HOW TO GROW YOUR HERBS FOR BEGINNERS

Self-sufficient Herbalism Using
Medicinal Herbs and Natural Remedies

Rosy Gilbert

TABLE OF CONTENT

The process is soft enjoy the journey with smile and grateful heart

INTRODUCTION

The Healing Power of Plants: A Personal Journey

I remember the first time I walked through my grandmother's herb garden. The air was thick with the mingling scents of rosemary, lavender, and mint, each plant whispering secrets of ancient wisdom and healing. As a child, I watched in awe as she effortlessly transformed these humble leaves and roots into potent remedies, soothing our ailments and lifting our spirits. It was here, amidst the vibrant greenery and fragrant blooms, that my journey into the world of herbal medicine began.

Years later, facing a barrage of stress and health challenges, I found myself yearning for the simplicity and efficacy of those natural remedies. Modern medicine, with its array of pills and synthetic solutions, felt impersonal and often brought a slew of unwanted side effects. I began to wonder if the answer to my wellness woes lay not in the pharmacy, but in the earth. Thus, I embarked on a mission to rediscover the healing power of plants, cultivating my own medicine right in my backyard.

This book is the culmination of that journey. It's a guide born from years of research, experimentation, and a profound respect for nature's pharmacy. Whether you're a seasoned gardener or a complete novice, my hope is that you'll find inspiration and practical advice within these pages, empowering you to take control of your health in the most natural and rewarding way possible.

Why Grow Your Own Medicine?

In a world where health crises are rampant and pharmaceutical solutions are often out of reach or fraught with side effects, many people are turning back to nature for answers. Growing your own herbal medicine offers a multitude of benefits that go beyond just the physical act of gardening. Here's why this practice can be life-changing:

1. **Health and Wellness**: Herbal remedies provide a holistic approach to health, addressing not just the symptoms but the root causes of ailments. Plants like echinacea, chamomile, and turmeric have been used for centuries to boost immunity, reduce inflammation, and promote overall well-being.

2. **Self-Sufficiency**: In an era of rising healthcare costs and uncertain access to medical care, having a personal supply of medicinal plants is empowering. You become less reliant on external

sources and can make informed decisions about your health.

3. **Sustainability**: Growing your own medicine is an environmentally friendly practice. It reduces your carbon footprint, minimizes waste from packaging, and promotes biodiversity in your garden.

4. **Connection to Nature**: Gardening has been shown to have therapeutic effects, reducing stress and enhancing mental clarity. The act of nurturing plants, watching them grow, and using them to heal yourself and your loved ones fosters a deep connection to the natural world.

5. **Economic Benefits**: Herbal medicine can be a cost-effective alternative to conventional drugs. Once established, your garden can provide a continuous supply of remedies, saving you money in the long run.

However, embarking on this journey is not without its challenges. Here are some common problems people face when growing their own herbal medicine, along with solutions to overcome them:

1. **Lack of Knowledge**: Many beginners feel overwhelmed by the sheer volume of information about herbal medicine. Solution: This book breaks down the process into manageable steps, providing clear, practical guidance on everything from soil preparation to harvesting.

2. **Limited Space**: Urban dwellers or those with small yards might think they don't have enough space to grow herbs. Solution: Learn about container gardening, vertical gardens, and selecting compact plant varieties suited for limited spaces.

3. **Time Constraints**: Busy lifestyles can make it hard to dedicate time to gardening. Solution: Discover low-maintenance herbs and efficient gardening techniques that fit into even the busiest schedules.

4. **Unpredictable Climate**: Weather can be a major factor affecting plant growth. Solution: Find out which herbs are best suited for your climate and learn how to create microclimates or use indoor gardening setups.

5. **Pest and Disease Management**: Dealing with pests and diseases can be daunting. Solution: Learn organic and sustainable methods for protecting your plants without resorting to harmful chemicals.

CHAPTER 1: INTRODUCTION TO HERBAL MEDICINE

The History and Benefits of Herbal Remedies

Often considered the forerunner of contemporary pharmacology, herbal therapy has a long and illustrious history that stretches back thousands of years. Civilizations across the globe, from the ancient Egyptians to the indigenous tribes of the Americas, have relied on the healing power of plants to treat a wide array of ailments. This rich tradition of using natural remedies is not only a testament to the efficacy of herbs but also highlights the deep connection between humans and nature.

The history of herbal medicine can be traced back to ancient texts such as the Ebers Papyrus from Egypt, which documents over 700 plant-based remedies used around 1550 BCE. Similarly, traditional Chinese medicine, with its extensive pharmacopeia recorded in the "Shennong Ben Cao Jing" around 2800 BCE, illustrates the comprehensive understanding ancient cultures had of botanical therapeutics. The Ayurvedic texts from India, dating back to 1500 BCE, also showcase an elaborate system of herbal treatments that continue to be used today.

Throughout history, herbs have been used not only to treat common illnesses but also to promote overall well-being and prevent disease. For instance, willow bark, used by the ancient Greeks and Native Americans, is the natural precursor to aspirin, providing pain relief and reducing inflammation. Garlic, celebrated in ancient Egyptian and Roman cultures, was used for its antibacterial properties and to boost cardiovascular health. These examples underline the significant role herbal medicine has played in shaping human health practices.

The benefits of herbal remedies are manifold. Firstly, they offer a natural alternative to synthetic drugs, often with fewer side effects. Unlike many modern pharmaceuticals, which can cause adverse reactions, herbs tend to work more gently with the body's natural processes. Additionally, herbal remedies are often more affordable and accessible, particularly for individuals in remote areas without easy access to modern healthcare facilities.

Furthermore, the holistic nature of herbal medicine addresses not just the symptoms but also the root causes of ailments. By focusing on overall health and balance, herbal treatments can enhance the body's ability to heal itself. For example, adaptogenic herbs like ashwagandha and rhodiola help the body manage stress and restore equilibrium, thereby improving resilience to various stressors.

Understanding How Herbal Medicine Works

To appreciate the efficacy of herbal medicine, it is crucial to understand how it works within the body. At its core, herbal medicine harnesses the pharmacological properties of plants to promote health and treat diseases. Each herb contains a complex array of bioactive compounds, including alkaloids, flavonoids, tannins, and glycosides, which interact with the body in unique ways to produce therapeutic effects.

The action of herbal remedies can be broken down into several key mechanisms. Firstly, herbs can provide direct pharmacological effects through their active constituents. For instance, the alkaloids in the herb goldenseal have strong antimicrobial properties, making it effective in treating infections. Similarly, the saponins in licorice root exhibit anti-inflammatory and immune-boosting effects, which can help alleviate symptoms of colds and flu.

Secondly, herbs can modulate physiological processes by supporting the body's natural functions. Adaptogens like ginseng and holy basil work by regulating the adrenal glands, helping the body adapt to stress and maintain homeostasis. This modulation is often more gentle and balanced compared to the immediate but sometimes harsh effects of synthetic drugs.

Another important aspect of herbal medicine is its synergistic nature. Herbs often contain multiple active compounds that work together to enhance their overall effect. This synergy can improve efficacy and reduce potential side effects. For example, the combination of different compounds in echinacea not only boosts the immune system but also provides anti-inflammatory and antiviral benefits, making it a powerful ally in fighting infections.

Moreover, herbal medicine places a strong emphasis on individualization and holistic treatment. Rather than concentrating only on treating specific symptoms, practitioners take into account the full individual, including their physical, emotional, and mental health. This approach ensures that treatment plans are tailored to the specific needs of each individual, promoting optimal health and wellness.

In addition to understanding the pharmacodynamics of herbs, it is essential to recognize the importance of quality and proper usage. The efficacy of herbal remedies depends significantly on the quality of the herbs used. Factors such as the plant's growing conditions, the timing of harvest, and the methods of preparation and storage all impact the potency and effectiveness of the final product. Therefore, sourcing high-quality herbs and preparing them correctly is vital for achieving the desired therapeutic outcomes.

Lastly, integrating herbal medicine with modern healthcare can provide comprehensive and complementary treatment options. While herbal remedies can be highly effective on their own, they can also be used alongside conventional treatments to enhance overall efficacy and improve patient outcomes. For instance, using turmeric to manage inflammation can complement standard anti-inflammatory medications, potentially allowing for lower doses and reducing the risk of side effects.

CHAPTER 2: GETTING STARTED WITH HERBAL GARDENING

Planning Your Medicinal Herb Garden

Embarking on the journey of herbal gardening is both exciting and rewarding. A well-thought-out plan is the cornerstone of a successful medicinal herb garden. Here's how to get started:

Understanding Your Goals

Before you dig into the soil, it's essential to define your goals. Are you looking to grow herbs for general wellness, specific ailments, or culinary purposes? Understanding your primary objectives will guide your selection of herbs and influence your garden's design.

Researching Medicinal Herbs

Take the time to research various medicinal herbs. Each herb has unique growing requirements, medicinal properties, and uses. Popular medicinal herbs include:

- **Echinacea**: Boosts the immune system.

- **Lavender**: Known for its calming effects.

- **Chamomile**: Helps with digestion and sleep.

- **Peppermint**: Soothes digestive issues.

Create a list of herbs that align with your goals and are suitable for your climate.

Designing Your Garden Layout

A well-designed garden layout not only looks beautiful but also promotes healthy growth. Consider the following elements when planning your garden:

- **Zones**: Divide your garden into zones based on the needs of different plants. For example, place sun-loving herbs in the sunniest spot and shade-tolerant ones in areas with partial shade.

- **Paths**: Create paths to easily access your plants for watering, weeding, and harvesting.

- **Companion Planting**: Some herbs thrive when planted next to specific companions. For instance, basil grows well alongside tomatoes and helps repel pests.

Sketch out a rough layout of your garden, keeping in mind the mature size of each plant to avoid overcrowding.

Choosing the Right Location and Containers

The location of your medicinal herb garden plays a crucial role in the success of your plants. Whether you have a sprawling backyard or a small balcony, here are some tips to choose the right spot and containers:

Finding the Ideal Location

When selecting a location for your herb garden, consider the following factors:

• **Sunlight**: Most medicinal herbs require at least 6-8 hours of direct sunlight each day. Select an area that gets lots of sunshine.

• **Soil Quality**: A flourishing garden starts with healthy soil. Verify that the soil has enough drainage and is rich in organic materials. Raised beds or containers are good options if the soil in your yard is poor.

• **Water Access**: Your herbs will need regular watering, especially during dry spells. Choose a location near a water source to make watering easier.

Selecting Containers

Container gardening is a great choice if you have limited space or would rather take a more flexible approach to gardening. When choosing containers, keep the following in mind:

- **Size**: Select plant pots that will hold your plants when they reach maturity. A container that is at least 12 inches deep is required for most herbs.

  o **Material**: There are many different types of containers, such as clay, plastic, and wood. Each has benefits and drawbacks:

o **Plastic**: It is lightweight and has good moisture retention, although it can heat up rapidly in the sun.

o **Clay**: Although it looks nice and has sufficient drainage, it dries out easily.

- **Wood**: aesthetically beautiful and effective in retaining moisture, but may need to be treated to avoid rot.

- **Drainage**: Make sure the containers you choose have openings for drainage in order to avoid waterlogging, which can cause root rot.

Creating the Right Environment

Regardless of where you choose to grow your herbs, it's important to provide the ideal environment:

- **Soil Preparation**: Use premium potting mix for container and in-ground gardening. Use compost to increase the soil's structure and fertility.

- **Mulching**: Mulch the area surrounding your plants to retain moisture, keep weeds out of the way, and control soil temperature.

- **Watering**: Water your herbs often and deeply, but don't overdo it. In general, herbs appreciate circumstances that are somewhat dry in between watering.

Getting Started

You're prepared to begin planting your medical herb garden now that you've designed it, selected the ideal spot, and selected containers. Remember that meticulous planning and preparation are the cornerstones of a successful herbal garden. Your garden will thrive with time and effort, giving you an abundant supply of therapeutic herbs for many years to come.

CHAPTER 3: SOIL AND COMPOST MASTERY

Understanding the soil, the building block of a healthy garden, is the first step towards growing your own therapeutic herbs. Soil is a living environment that sustains plant life, not just dirt. This chapter will cover the science and art of creating the ideal soil for growing medicinal herbs as well as the importance of organic compost in growing a strong, fruitful garden.

Like all plants, medicinal herbs have unique soil requirements that, when satisfied, may result in lush, powerful plants full of the chemicals that give them their therapeutic value. The following are the essential procedures for creating the ideal soil for your herb garden:

1. **Understanding Soil Composition**: Air, water, organic stuff, and minerals make up soil. Its texture, structure, and fertility are influenced by the proportions of these elements. Loamy soil is the best type of soil for growing most medicinal plants since it has a good mixture of clay, silt, and sand. In order to avoid root rot and other water-related problems, this kind of soil lets excess water drain away while retaining moisture and nutrients.

2. **Soil Testing**: It's important to test your soil to find out its pH and nutrient content before planting. The majority of therapeutic herbs prefer neutral to

slightly acidic soil (pH 6.0 to 7.0). For a more thorough study, you can utilize a home testing kit or submit a sample to your neighborhood agricultural extension office. You may determine what amendments are necessary to maximize soil health by conducting a soil test.

3. **Amending the Soil**: To produce the perfect growth conditions, you might need to modify your soil based on the findings of the soil test. Typical soil additives consist of:

   - **Organic Matter**: Water retention, nutritional content, and soil structure are all improved by adding compost, leaf mold, or well-rotted manure.

   - **Lime or Sulfur**: Soil pH can be adjusted with these. While sulfur reduces pH (making soil more acidic), lime raises pH (making soil less acidic).

4. **Mineral Additions**: Important minerals like phosphorus and potassium are added via greensand, bone meal, and rock phosphate.

5. **Soil Aeration and Drainage**: Root health depends on adequate soil aeration. Compacted soil decreases the amount of available oxygen and limits root development. Consider double digging or using a broadfork to loosen the soil without turning it over in order to maintain the soil's structure and increase aeration. If your soil is thick clay, you should also add sand or perlite to guarantee proper drainage.

6. **Mulching**: Mulching controls temperature, inhibits weed growth, and helps keep the soil wet. Make use of organic mulches, such as wood chips, straw, or shredded leaves, since they will break down and enrich the soil with organic matter.

The Importance of Organic Compost

An organic garden's foundation is compost made of organic materials. It improves microbial activity, enriches the soil, and offers a slow-release supply of vital nutrients. Here's why cultivating therapeutic herbs need organic compost:

1. **Nutrient-Rich**: Plants require a balanced combination of nutrients, which compost is full of. Compost distributes nutrients gradually, as opposed to synthetic fertilizers, so there is a continuous supply throughout time. This gradual release lessens the chance of over fertilization, which can damage plants, and stops nutrient leaking.

2. **Improves Soil Structure**: Compost improves soil texture, increasing the friability of heavy clay soils and improving the moisture and nutrient retention of sandy soils. It contributes to the formation of a crumbly soil structure that is favorable for root development.

3. **Increases Water Retention**: Compost helps the soil retain more water by enhancing its structure. This is particularly crucial for medicinal plants, many of which need constant moisture yet decay easily if left wet.

4. **Promotes Beneficial Microbes**: Beneficial microorganisms that support plant development, disease prevention, and nutrient cycling abound in healthy soil. These microorganisms find a home and a food supply in compost, which improves soil fertility and plant health.

5. **Reduces Waste and Recycles Nutrients**: Yard trash, food leftovers, and other organic items may be composted to recycle their nutrients back into the soil and keep them out of the landfill. This eco-friendly method lessens your environmental impact while simultaneously improving your landscape.

Creating Your Own Compost

1. Composting is easy to do yourself, and you may do it in a backyard container or a makeshift pile. Take a look at this quick tutorial to get you started:

2. **Collect Organic Materials**: assemble a mixture of brown (high in carbon) and green (rich in nitrogen) elements. Kitchen trash, coffee grounds, and grass clippings are considered greens, whereas cardboard, leaves, and straw are considered browns.

3. **Build the Pile**: To balance carbon and nitrogen, alternate layers of brown and green. Aim for a brown-to-green ratio of around three to one. Make sure every layer is damp but not drenched.

4. **Maintain the Pile**: To promote faster decomposition and aeration, turn the pile frequently. To keep the pile damp, add water as needed to keep it at the consistency of wet sponge.

5. **Harvest the Compost**: Your compost is going to be ready in several months to a year. It smells earthy and should be crumbly and black. Once you sift it to get rid of any big, partially decomposed bits, you may use it on your garden.

CHAPTER 4: PROPAGATION TECHNIQUES FOR MEDICINAL PLANTS

Seed Starting Basics

Planting medicinal plants from seed may be a very fulfilling experience. It gives you the opportunity to choose the exact types you like and gives you a sense of satisfaction as you see your plants develop from little seeds into mature, useful herbs. Here's a thorough how-to tutorial to get you going:

Selecting Seeds

Selecting premium seeds is the first stage in the seed starting process. Seek out trustworthy vendors with expertise in medicinal herbs. Observe the germination rates and any particular guidelines that may be given. Certain medicinal plants could require special care or take longer to germinate.

Preparing Your Soil   start here

The soil has to be ready for seed to begin to sprout. Use a seed starting mix that is light and easily drained. You may manufacture your own mix using equal parts vermiculite, perlite, and peat moss, or you can purchase one already made. Early seedlings shouldn't be planted in garden soil since it might be quite heavy and contaminated.

Planting Seeds

1. **Containers:** Use reusable containers like seed starting trays, egg cartons, or small pots. To prevent waterlogging, make sure there are drainage outlets.

2. **Sowing Seeds:** as specified in the packaging that came with your seeds. Generally speaking, seeds need to be planted two to three times deeply than they are wide. Some seeds need sunlight to germinate, thus they should be sown on the top of the soil.

3. **Watering:** To prevent the seeds from moving, lightly mist them with a water spray bottle. Ensure that the ground is consistently damp but not drenched.

Providing the Right Conditions

1. **Light:** Most seedlings need a lot of sunlight to germinate. Should natural light prove inadequate, grow lights may provide illumination for up to 12 to 16 hours per day.

2. **Temperature:** Temperature: 65 to 75°F (18 to 24°C) is usually the ideal temperature range for seeds to germinate. Use a seedling heat pad if you must maintain a steady temperature.

3. **Humidity:** You may use a plastic dome or plastic wrap to stabilize the humidity levels in your seed trays. Take off the cover as soon as the seedlings sprout to prevent fungal diseases.

Transplanting Seedlings

Your seedlings are prepared for transplantation once they have produced a few genuine leaves. To help them become more resilient, expose them to outside conditions progressively over the course of a week. When you move them into larger pots or directly onto your garden bed, make sure they are positioned appropriately to accommodate their mature size.

Advanced Propagation: Cuttings, Division, and Layering

While starting from seeds is a popular way, more advanced techniques like as layering, dividing, and taking cuttings can ensure that you are growing exact clones of the desired plants. How to become proficient using these methods:

Cuttings

Propagation of cuttings from a wide range of medicinal plants is simple. With this technique, a portion of the plant is chopped off, and the roots spread out on their own.

1. **Selecting the Cutting:** Choose sturdy, nonflowering stems. Slice off 4-6 inches just below a leaf node.

2. **Preparing the Cutting:** To promote the growth of roots, remove the lower leaves and immerse the cut end in rooting hormone.

3. **Planting the Cutting:** Put the cutting in a pot with a suitable drainage system filled with a perlite and peat mixture. Firm the dirt around the stem and then give it plenty of water.

4. **Providing the Right Environment:** Keep the cutting somewhere warm, muggy, and with indirect light. You may help preserve humidity by covering with a plastic bag. Mist often to keep the soil wet but not soggy.

5. **Transplanting:** In a few weeks, when the cutting has taken root, transplant it into a larger pot or directly into the garden.

Division

1. Plants that grow in clusters or with spreading roots can proliferate through division. It's a great way to give old plants new life.

2. **Identifying Candidates for Division:** Some plants that are ideal choices for division are echinacea, lemon balm, and mint.

3. **Digging Up the Plant:** Take great care to remove the entire plant without damaging the root system.

4. **Dividing the Plant:** Using a sharp knife or garden spade, divide the root mass into sections. A piece of the root system and numerous healthy shoots should be present in each region.

5. **Replanting:** When you immediately transplant the divisions, make sure they are planted at the same depth as when they were originally growing. Give the soil frequent dampness and lots of water until the plants are well-established.

Layering

A branch of the plant is encouraged to root while it is still connected to the parent plant when it is propagated by layering.

1. **Selecting a Branch:** Select a branch that can be bent all the way to the ground without breaking; it should be strong and flexible.

2. **Preparing the Branch:** Remove the leaves from a 6 to 12 inch section of the branch. To encourage the growth of roots, make a small incision at the bottom of the stem.

3. **Securing the Branch:** You should be able to see the tip of the branch as you bury the damaged part in the earth. Use a U-shaped pin or a rock to keep the branch in contact with the ground.

4. **Caring for the Layering:** Keep the soil moist while you wait for the roots to develop. It could take several months to finish this. Once roots have

taken hold, cut the young plant off from the parent and transplant it to the new location.

CHAPTER 5: ESSENTIAL MEDICINAL HERBS TO GROW

People have regarded medicinal plants for their holistic benefits and healing abilities for eons. Not only can these plants provide fresh, organic ingredients for your treatments, but growing them in your own yard fosters a stronger contact with the natural world. The top ten important medicinal herbs will be covered in this chapter, along with comprehensive growing and care guidelines for each one. xxxx

Top 10 Must-Have Medicinal Herbs

1. **Echinacea (Echinacea purpurea)**

   o **Uses:** strengthens the immune system, lessens flu and cold symptoms, and speeds up the healing of wounds.

Growing Tips: Echinacea favors soil that drains well and full sun. In the spring, sow seeds or seedlings. Use moderate watering and make sure there's adequate airflow to avoid fungal infections.

2. **Lavender (Lavandula angustifolia)**

   o **Uses:** eases skin irritations, lowers tension and anxiety, and enhances the quality of sleep.

   o **Growing Tips:** Full sun and sandy, somewhat alkaline soil are ideal for lavender growth. To promote bushy growth and more blossoms, plant in the spring or fall and trim often.

3. **Peppermint (Mentha piperita)**

   o **Uses:** reduces headaches, eases intestinal problems, and freshens breath.

   Growing Tips: Partially shaded, well-drained soil that is wet is ideal for peppermint growth. Because it's an invasive plant, you might want to use root barriers or containers.

4. **Chamomile (Matricaria chamomilla)**

- o **Uses:** contains anti-inflammatory qualities, assists with digestion, and encourages relaxation.

    Growing Tips: Chamomile likes soil that drains well and full light. Plant seeds in the spring and trim out seedlings to make sure there's enough airflow. When flowers are completely open, harvest them.

5. **Lemon Balm (Melissa officinalis)**

    - o **Uses:** enhances mood, eases tension and anxiety, and promotes intestinal health.

    - o **Growing Tips:** Lemon balm grows best in well-drained soil with full or partial shade. Water often and plant in the spring. To keep the plant from getting too lanky, prune it.

6. **Aloe Vera (Aloe barbadensis miller)**

    - o **Uses:** relieves burns and skin irritations, promotes the healing of wounds, and is good for the digestive system.

- o **Growing Tips:** Aloe Vera needs sandy soil that drains properly and full light. Water plants sparingly whether they are planted in the ground or in containers. When watering, allow the soil to dry fully between applications.

7. **Calendula (Calendula officinalis)**

   - o **Uses:** heals cuts, lowers inflammation, and calms skin issues.

   - o **Growing Tips:** Calendula prefers full sun to partial shade and well-drained soil. Sow seeds in the spring or fall, and deadhead spent flowers to encourage continuous blooming.

8. **Thyme (Thymus vulgaris)**

   - o **Uses:** Supports respiratory health, has antibacterial properties, and aids digestion.

- o **Growing Tips:** Thyme thrives in full sun and well-drained soil. Plant seeds or cuttings in the spring, and water sparingly. Trim regularly to promote new growth and prevent woody stems.

9. **Ginger (Zingiber officinale)**

- o **Uses:** Relieves nausea, aids digestion, and reduces inflammation.

- o **Growing Tips:** Ginger prefers partial shade and rich, moist soil. Plant rhizomes in the spring, and water regularly. Mulch to shield roots and hold in moisture.

10. **Turmeric (Curcuma longa)**

- o **Uses:** Reduces inflammation, supports joint health, and boosts the immune system.

- o **Growing Tips:** Turmeric thrives in partial shade and well-drained, fertile soil. Plant rhizomes in the spring, and water consistently. When the leaves begin to yellow and wither back, harvest them.

Growing and Caring for Each Herb

Echinacea: Sow echinacea seeds or seedlings in well-drained soil in a sunny location. Water sparingly, letting the soil dry up in between applications. In order to promote additional blooms and stop self-seeding, deadhead wasted blossoms. When the plant is two or three years old, harvest the roots in the fall.

Lavender: When growing lavender, pick a sunny spot with well-drained, somewhat alkaline soil. Plants should be spaced 12 to 18 inches apart to promote proper airflow. To reshape the plant and get rid of dead wood, prune in the spring. To get the finest scent and oil content, harvest blossoms right before they open completely.

Peppermint: Plant peppermint on soil that is wet and well-drained, with moderate shade. To reduce its invasiveness, think about growing it in containers. To keep the soil damp but not soggy, water it often. To promote continued development, harvest leaves as needed, but do not take more than one-third of the plant at a time.

Chamomile: Plant chamomile seeds in a sunny spot with well-drained soil. Plant seedlings thinly to provide proper air circulation and avoid crowding. Drink plenty of water, especially in the dry months. When the blooms are completely open, harvest them and dry them so you may use them later in teas and infusions.

Lemon Balm: Plant lemon balm in well-drained soil in a sunny or partly shady spot. Sow seedlings thinly to avoid crowding and to provide proper ventilation.. Be sure to stay hydrated, especially during the arid months. When the blooms are completely open, harvest them and dry them so you may use them later in teas and infusions.

Aloe Vera: Aloe vera can be planted in the ground in a sunny position or in containers with well-drained, sandy soil. Use water sparingly, letting the soil dry up entirely in between applications. To stop root rot, don't overwater. Remove outer leaves as needed, trimming toward the root.

Calendula: Plant calendula seeds in a sunny spot with well-drained soil. Be sure to stay hydrated, especially during the arid months. Remove spent petals to promote ongoing flowering. When completely opened, gather flowers for use in salves and ointments, either fresh or dried.

Thyme: Thyme should be planted in well-drained soil in a sunny area. Plants should be spaced 12 inches apart to promote proper airflow. Water seldom since thyme likes dry weather. To encourage new growth and avoid woody stems, trim often. Harvest leaves as needed for both medicinal and culinary purposes.

Ginger: Plant the roots of ginger in well-drained, slightly shaded soil. To maintain constant moisture in the soil, water it often. Mulch to keep moisture in and shield roots from changes in temperature. After the plant's leaves have withered and become yellow, harvest the rhizomes of ginger.

Turmeric: Plant the rhizomes of turmeric in a somewhat shaded area with well-drained, healthy soil. Water regularly to maintain soil moisture. Mulch to shield roots and hold in moisture. Turmeric should be harvested eight to ten months after planting, or when the leaves begin to turn yellow and wither back. Adding these healing herbs to your garden will improve your health and well-being while strengthening your bond with the natural world. Every plant has a special set of advantages, and you may take natural control of your health by learning how to cultivate and take care of them.

CHAPTER 6: GARDEN MAINTENANCE AND TROUBLESHOOTING

Care and attention to detail are necessary for the ongoing maintenance of a healthy herbal garden. Effective garden care guarantees that your medicinal plants flourish and provide you with a steady supply of natural cures. This includes routine watering and controlling pests and illnesses. This chapter will cover typical pests and illnesses that may impact your herbal garden as well as organic ways to maintain the health and robustness of your plants.

Common Pests and Diseases in Herbal Gardens

1. Herbal gardens are no different from other gardens in that pests and illnesses provide problems to gardeners. A fruitful garden requires early detection of these problems and knowledge on how to address them. The following are some of the most typical illnesses and pests you may run into:

2. **Aphids**: These small, soft-bodied insects suck the sap from plants, causing leaves to yellow and curl. Additionally, aphids can spread illness among plants.

   - **Solution**: Introduce beneficial insects like ladybugs, which feed on aphids. Alternatively, use a homemade spray of water mixed with a few drops of dish soap to dislodge and kill them.

3. **Caterpillars**: While some caterpillars transform into beautiful butterflies, others can decimate your plants by eating the leaves.

   - **Solution**: Handpick caterpillars from your plants and relocate them. Using neem oil or Bacillus thuringiensis (Bt) can also help control their population.

4. **Powdery Mildew**: This fungal disease appears as a white, powdery coating on leaves, stems, and

buds, inhibiting photosynthesis and weakening the plant.

- **Solution**: Improve air circulation around your plants by spacing them properly and pruning any overcrowded areas. Spray affected plants with a mixture of baking soda, water, and a few drops of liquid soap.

5. **Spider Mites**: These tiny arachnids thrive in hot, dry conditions and cause stippling on leaves, eventually leading to leaf drop.

- **Solution**: Increase humidity around your plants and regularly mist them with water. Introduce predatory mites or spray plants with insecticidal soap.

6. **Leaf Miners**: These pests burrow into leaves, creating winding trails that can stunt plant growth.

- **Solution**: Remove and destroy affected leaves. Use floating row covers to prevent adult insects from laying eggs on your plants.

7. **Root Rot**: Caused by overwatering and poor drainage, root rot leads to the decay of plant roots, resulting in wilting and yellowing of foliage.

   o **Solution**: Ensure your garden has well-draining soil and avoid overwatering. If root rot is detected, remove affected plants and improve soil drainage.

8. **Rust**: This fungal disease causes orange or yellow spots on the underside of leaves, eventually leading to leaf drop.

   o **Solution**: Remove and destroy affected leaves. Apply organic fungicides like sulfur or copper-based sprays.

Organic Solutions For Garden Problems

Maintaining an organic herbal garden means avoiding synthetic chemicals and opting for natural solutions to address garden problems. Here are some effective organic methods to keep your garden healthy:

1. **Companion Planting**: Plant herbs and flowers that repel pests or attract beneficial insects. For example, marigolds deter nematodes, while basil can repel flies and mosquitoes.

2. **Neem Oil**: Extracted from the neem tree, this oil acts as a natural pesticide and fungicide. It disrupts the life cycle of insects and prevents fungal spores from germinating.

3. **Diatomaceous Earth**: Made from fossilized algae, diatomaceous earth is a fine powder that can be sprinkled around plants to deter crawling insects like slugs and beetles. It works by dehydrating their exoskeletons.

4. **Homemade Sprays**: Create your own pest control sprays using common household ingredients. A mixture of garlic, chili peppers, and water can

repel insects, while a solution of milk and water can combat powdery mildew.

5. **Beneficial Insects**: Introduce predators such as ladybugs, lacewings, and predatory mites to your garden. These insects feed on common pests like aphids, spider mites, and caterpillars.

6. **Composting**: Regularly add compost to your soil to improve its structure, fertility, and microbial activity. Healthy soil produces stronger plants that are more resistant to pests and diseases.

7. **Mulching**: Apply a layer of organic mulch around your plants to retain moisture, regulate soil temperature, and suppress weed growth. Mulch also helps prevent soil-borne diseases by reducing water splashes onto leaves.

8. **Crop Rotation**: Rotate your crops each season to prevent the buildup of pests and diseases that target specific plants. This method aids in preserving the fertility and structure of the soil.

9. **Handpicking**: Handpicking is a quick and efficient way to get rid of bigger pests like beetles and caterpillars. Check your plants frequently, and get rid of any pests that are obvious.

10. **Biological Controls**: Use naturally occurring organisms to control pests. For instance, Bacillus thuringiensis (Bt) is a soil-dwelling bacterium that targets caterpillars, while Trichoderma fungi can suppress soil-borne diseases.

CHAPTER 7: HARVESTING YOUR HERBS

When and How to Harvest Different Herbs

To guarantee that you obtain the most potency and benefit from your plants, it is important to harvest herbs at the appropriate time. Every herb has a best time to harvest it, which is usually when the plant's active ingredients and essential oils are at their best. The ideal seasons and techniques for harvesting some of the most widely used medicinal plants are discussed here.

1. **Basil**

   o **When to Harvest:** Basil should be harvested just before it flowers when the leaves are at their most flavorful and aromatic.

2. **How to Harvest:** Use sharp scissors or garden shears to cut the stem about 1/4 inch above a pair of leaves or a branching point. This promotes

bushier growth and increased leaf production on the plant.

Chamomile

- o **When to Harvest:** Harvest chamomile when the flowers are fully open but before they begin to wither.

- o **How to Harvest:** Gently pinch the flower heads off the stems. You can also use a chamomile rake or a similar tool to make harvesting faster.

3. **Lavender**

- o **When to Harvest:** The best time to harvest lavender is when the flowers are just starting to open, as this is when the essential oil content is highest.

- o **How to Harvest:** Cut the stems just above the leaves using sharp scissors or shears, and gather the stems into small bundles.

4. Mint

- When to Harvest: Mint can be harvested just before it flowers for the best flavor.

- How to Harvest: Cut the stems down to about an inch above the soil. Frequent harvesting prevents the plant from growing lanky and promotes fresh growth.

5. Rosemary

- When to Harvest: Rosemary can be harvested year-round, but it's best just before the plant blooms.

- How to Harvest: Snip the sprigs of rosemary with sharp scissors or pruning shears. Avoid cutting more than a third of the plant at a time to ensure it remains healthy.

6. Echinacea

o **When to Harvest:** Harvest echinacea flowers when they are in full bloom.

o **How to Harvest:** Cut the flowers off the stems and leave a few inches of stem attached. The roots can also be harvested in the fall after the plant has gone dormant.

7. **Calendula**

o **When to Harvest:** Calendula should be harvested when the flowers are fully open.

o **How to Harvest:** Pinch or cut the flower heads off the plant. Regular harvesting encourages more blooms.

Drying and Storing Your Harvest

Correct drying and storage are essential if you want to preserve the potency and effectiveness of your harvested herbs. This is a comprehensive guide on drying and storing your herbs correctly.

1. **Drying Your Herbs**

   o **Air Drying:** This is the most conventional approach and is effective for herbs such as thyme and rosemary that have little moisture content. Sort the herbs into little bunches and place them upside down in a place that is dry, dark, and has good ventilation. One to two weeks may pass throughout this process.

   o **Using a Dehydrator:** With a dehydrator, you may get faster results. Arrange the herbs on the trays in a single layer and preheat the dehydrator to a low 95–115°F. For plants like mint and basil that have a high moisture content, this technique works particularly well.

   o **Oven Drying:** Oven Drying: Place the herbs in an equal layer on a baking sheet, then set the oven to the lowest setting with the door slightly ajar. Check often to prevent over-drying. Although speedier, this approach needs careful observation.

2. Storing Your Herbs

- **Containers**: Store the herbs in airtight jars after they have fully dried. The best containers are glass jars with tight-fitting lids because they keep light and moisture from deteriorating the herbs.

- **Labeling:** Put the herb's name and the harvest date on the label of each container. You can monitor the freshness of your herbs with the use of this.

- **Storage Location:** The containers should be kept somewhere dry, dark, and cold. Herbs might lose their quality over time if they are kept in direct sunlight or close to heat sources.

CHAPTER 8: MAKING HERBAL PREPARATIONS

We go into the craft and science of creating herbal concoctions in this chapter, turning the herbs you've planted and collected into powerful cures. Anyone hoping to maximize the therapeutic benefits of their plants must comprehend these techniques. To make sure you have a complete arsenal for herbal therapy, we'll go over both fundamental and sophisticated procedures.

Basic Herbal Preparations: Teas, Tinctures, and Infusions

Teas: The Simplicity of Herbal Healing

One of the easiest and most convenient methods to benefit from the properties of medicinal plants is through herbal teas, or tisanes. Here's how to get them ready:

1. **Choosing Your Herbs**: Choose between dried or fresh herbs. Popular options include ginger's anti-inflammatory qualities, peppermint for digestion, and chamomile for relaxation.

2. **Brewing:** Use a teaspoon of dried or a tablespoon of fresh herbs for every cup of tea. Cover the herbs with boiling water, then let steep for five to ten minutes. Take a strain and relish.

3. **Adjusting for Strength**: Use extra herbs or soak it longer for a stronger tea. If desired, sweeten with honey or lemon.

Tinctures: Concentrated Herbal Power

Strong liquid extracts known as tinctures are created by immersing plants in glycerin or alcohol. They have a lengthy shelf life and are quite concentrated.

1. **Selecting Herbs and Solvents**: Select your herbs and the proper solvent. The most popular type of alcohol is vodka or brandy, however glycerin may be used to make tinctures without alcohol.

2. **Preparation**: Prepare by putting one-third of the dried herbs or half of the chopped fresh herbs into a jar. Make sure the herbs are well submerged by pouring your solvent over them. Store the sealed jar in a cool, dark place with occasional shaking for four to six weeks.

3. **Straining and Bottling**: The mixture should be strained using cheesecloth or a fine mesh strainer after four to six weeks. Label and store the liquid after bottling it into opaque glass containers.

Infusions: Extracting the Goodness

Similar to teas, infusions are made with harder plant components like roots and bark and are usually stronger and steeped longer.

1. **Herbs and Water Ratio**: For every quart of water, use one ounce of dry herbs.

2. **Brewing:** Put the herbs in a pot or jar, cover with boiling water, and bring to a boil. Steep for a few hours or maybe overnight.

3. **Straining and Usage:** After straining the infusion, it is prepared for use. Infusion-based beverages can also be applied topically as washes or compresses.

Advanced Techniques: Salves, Syrups, and Capsules

Salves: Restorative Skin Ointments

Topically applied salves soothe and restore skin. They are semi-solid formulations.

1. **Infusing Oils**: Begin by soaking your herbs in an oil carrier (such as almond, coconut, or olive oil). Put herbs in a container and pour oil over it. Shake occasionally and let lie for a few weeks, or heat gently in a double boiler for a few hours.

2. **Straining and Mixing:** After the oil has been strained, add one ounce of melted beeswax for every cup of oil to a double boiler. Add essential oils if desired.

3. **Pouring and Cooling**: After filling tins or jars, allow the mixture to cool. You can now utilize your salve.

Syrups: Sweet Herbal Remedies

Herbal syrups blend the calming effects of sugar or honey with the therapeutic benefits of plants.

1. Preparing a Decoction: Half a pint of water should be lowered by simmering one ounce of herbs in it.

2. Adding Sweetener: Pour the decoction back into the saucepan after straining it. When the sugar or honey is added, boil it until it dissolves.

3. Storage: Transfer into sterile bottles and place them in the fridge. Use as a daily tonic or as needed for coughs and colds.

Capsules: Convenient Herbal Dosage

Capsules are an excellent way to take herbs when you need precise dosing or don't enjoy the taste of certain preparations.

1. **Grinding Herbs**: Grind dried herbs into a fine powder using a coffee grinder or mortar and pestle.

2. Filling Capsules: Pour the powdered herbs into empty capsules using a capsule maker. This ensures consistency and saves time.

3. **Storage and Use**: Store filled capsules in a cool, dark place. Follow recommended dosages based on the specific herb and individual needs.

CHAPTER 9: DOSAGE AND ADMINISTRATION OF HERBAL REMEDIES

Safe and Effective Dosage Guidelines

The right dose must be chosen for herbal treatments in order to ensure safety and efficacy. Herbal doses, in contrast to pharmaceutical dosages, can differ significantly based on the plant, the ailment being treated, and the individual's particular qualities. In order to guarantee that you give herbal treatments safely and successfully, we'll go over some general recommendations and concepts below.

1. Understanding Herb Potency and Concentration

Herbs can be found in tinctures, extracts, dried, fresh, and capsule form. An herb's potency might differ greatly depending on how it is prepared and in what form. For example, tinctures and extracts require lesser doses since they are more concentrated than dried or fresh plants. Always follow the instructions relevant to the herb and standardize your measurements.

2. Start Low and Go Slow Gradually increasing a little dose at first is a cornerstone of herbal treatment. This method reduces the possibility of negative effects while assisting in determining how your body will react to the herb. Keep an eye out for any changes in your health and modify the dosage as necessary.

3. Dosage by Age and Weight Take into account the patient's age and weight while using the herbal medicine. Lower doses are frequently needed for children, the elderly, and those with impaired health. A well-liked method that adjusts the adult dosage based on the weight of the youngster is called Clark's Rule.

4. Herb-Specific Dosage Recommendations The recommended dose for each plant varies. As an illustration:

- **Echinacea:** Twice a day, 300 mg of dry extract.

- **Ginger:** Two to three times a day, ingest 1-2 grams of fresh root or 250–500 mg of dried root.

- **Valerian:** Two hours before to going to bed, 400–900 mg of valerian extract.

For precise dose recommendations for any plant you take, speak with a qualified herbalist or dependable herbal sources.

Safety Precautions

- **Allergic Reactions:** Recognize any possible allergies. Take it slow at first and keep an eye out for any adverse reactions.

- **Interactions:** Certain herbs may not work well with other herbs or drugs. Investigate or speak with a medical professional to prevent negative interactions.

- **Pregnancy and Nursing:** Some herbs should not be used when nursing or pregnant. Always be sure that using herbs in these circumstances is safe.

Administering Herbal Remedies for Optimal Results

Correct use of herbal treatments might increase their effectiveness. To make sure you get the most out of your herbal therapies, consider the following recommended practices.

1. Choosing the Right Form Select the appropriate form of the herb based on the condition you are treating and your personal preference. For instance, teas are excellent for digestive issues, while tinctures may be better for systemic conditions like anxiety.

2. Timing and Frequency The timing of herbal administration can affect its efficacy. Some herbs work best when taken on an empty stomach, while others should be taken with food. Additionally, the frequency of dosage is important; some herbs require multiple doses throughout the day, while others are effective with a single dose.

Method of Preparation

- **Teas and Infusions:** Use boiling water for leaves, flowers, and soft stems. Steep for 10-15 minutes.

- **Decoctions:** Boil roots, bark, and seeds for 20-30 minutes to extract their medicinal properties.

- **Tinctures and Extracts:** Follow the recommended drops or milliliters, usually diluted in water.

Combining Herbs Combining herbs can enhance their effects through synergy. For example, combining peppermint with ginger can enhance digestive relief. However, be cautious and research potential interactions between herbs.

Record Keeping: Keep a journal of your herbal usage. Note the herb, dosage, frequency, and any observed effects. This practice helps in fine-tuning your herbal regimen and identifying any adverse reactions.

Adjusting Dosages Herbal remedies may require dosage adjustments based on individual response and changing conditions. Regularly assess the effectiveness of the treatment and make necessary adjustments.

Practical Tips for Administration

1. Measuring Accuracy Invest in a good set of measuring spoons, a kitchen scale, and a dropper for precise measurement of herbs, especially tinctures and extracts.

2. Flavor Enhancements Some herbs can be bitter or unpleasant in taste. Enhance the flavor with natural sweeteners like honey or stevia, or mix them with palatable herbs such as mint or licorice.

3. Incorporating into Daily Routine Make herbal administration a part of your daily routine. Set reminders if necessary and create a ritual around your herbal practice to ensure consistency.

4. Educate and Empower Educate yourself continuously about the herbs you use. Empower others by sharing your knowledge and experiences, fostering a community of informed herbal users.

CHAPTER 10: CREATING PERSONALIZED HERBAL REGIMENS

Tailoring Herbal Medicine to Your Needs

Developing individualized herbal regimens requires careful consideration of how various herbs might enhance your well-being and your particular set of health demands. Customizing herbal medicine to meet your requirements is a liberating experience that changes the way you view your health and fosters a closer bond with the natural world.

Assessing Your Health Needs

Assembling a customized herbal regimen starts with determining your medical needs. This entails a thorough assessment of your present state of health, taking into account any allergies, chronic diseases, or particular health objectives you may have. To learn more about your health and get advice on which herbs could be good for you, think about speaking with a trained herbalist or medical practitioner.

Selecting the Right Herbs

Choosing the appropriate herbs is the next step after determining your specific health needs. Herbs may treat a wide range of health problems and have diverse qualities. As an illustration:

- **Chamomile** is known for its calming effects and is great for anxiety and digestive issues.

- **Echinacea** is commonly used to boost the immune system and fight infections.

- **Ginger** is effective for nausea and inflammation.

- **Lavender** is great for encouraging sleep and relieving stress.

Research each herb to understand its benefits, potential side effects, and how it can be incorporated into your regimen. It's important to start with a small number of herbs to see how your body responds before adding more.

Formulating Your Regimen

When formulating your herbal regimen, consider the following:

- **Dosage**: The amount of herb you take is crucial. Dosages can vary based on the form of the herb (e.g., tincture, tea, capsule) and your individual needs.

- **Frequency**: Determine how often you need to take each herb. Some may be taken daily, while others are better suited for occasional use.

- **Combination**: Some herbs work synergistically, enhancing each other's effects. However, it's essential to understand which combinations are safe and effective.

An example of a personalized regimen might include a morning tea blend of chamomile and lavender for relaxation, a mid-day capsule of ginger for digestive support, and an evening tincture of echinacea to boost the immune system.

Monitoring and Adjusting

Your herbal regimen should be dynamic and adaptable. Regularly monitor your body's response to the herbs. Keep track of any changes in your symptoms, overall health, and any side effects you may experience. Adjust the dosages or combinations as needed, and don't hesitate to consult with a healthcare professional if you have any concerns.

Keeping a Herbal Medicine Journal

Maintaining a herbal medicine journal is an invaluable tool in your journey toward personalized herbal health. It helps you keep track of your regimen, monitor your progress, and make informed adjustments.

Starting Your Journal

Begin your herbal medicine journal by noting your initial health assessment. Include details such as:

- Your current health status and any specific conditions

- Your health goals

- Herbs you are starting with and their intended purposes

Daily Entries

Your daily entries should include:

- **Herbs Taken**: List the herbs you took that day, including the form (tea, tincture, capsule), dosage, and frequency.

- **Symptoms and Effects**: Note any changes in your symptoms, overall well-being, and any side effects.

- **Emotional and Mental State**: Herbal medicine not only affects the body but also the mind. Record your emotional and mental state to see if the herbs impact your mood, stress levels, or sleep patterns.

Weekly and Monthly Reviews

Periodically review your journal to identify patterns and trends. This review can help you understand how your body responds to the herbs over time and make necessary adjustments to your regimen. Consider the following in your reviews:

- Are there any improvements in your symptoms?

- Have you experienced any side effects?

- Are there any herbs that are particularly effective or ineffective?

Reflect and Adjust

Use your journal entries to reflect on your progress and make informed decisions about your regimen. If a particular herb is working well, you may want to continue with it or even increase its dosage. Conversely, if you notice any adverse effects, consider reducing the dosage or discontinuing the herb.

Consulting with Professionals

Sharing your herbal medicine journal with a healthcare professional or herbalist can provide them with valuable insights into your health journey. They can offer advice, suggest new herbs, or help you refine your regimen based on your documented experiences.

CHAPTER 11: BUILDING A COMMUNITY AROUND HERBAL MEDICINE

Sharing Knowledge and Resources

Sharing information and resources is the first step towards creating a community around herbal medicine. It is imperative that you understand that a community's power is derived from the combined expertise and support of its members as you set out on your journey. In addition to empowering others, imparting your knowledge of herbal medicine strengthens your own comprehension and promotes a spirit of unity and progress amongst you.

1. Starting with Friends and Family

Start by telling individuals closest to you about your interest. Discuss the advantages of herbal medicine and how it has improved your life with your loved ones. You might begin simply, showing them around your herb garden or sharing a few of your best herbal cures. This intimate touch frequently piques curiosity and intrigue, opening the door to more in-depth discussions.

2. Utilizing Social Media

Social networking sites are excellent resources for interacting with like-minded people and sharing information. Make a herbal medicine-focused blog, Facebook group, or Instagram account. Talk about your experiences, advice, and recipes. Videos, before-and-after pictures, and testimonials are examples of engaging material that may draw viewers and start conversations. Recall to engage your audience by answering their queries and remarks, since this fosters a feeling of community and trust.

3. Collaborating with Local Health Stores and Community Centers

Libraries, community centers, and health stores in the area frequently hold workshops and activities. Collaborate with these establishments to plan discussions, workshops, or Q&A sessions on herbal medicine. These locations offer a way to engage with people who might already be interested in natural health practices and reach a larger audience.

4. Creating Informative Materials

Create newsletters, leaflets, or booklets that include insightful information on herbal treatment. These documents can be given out at neighborhood gatherings, pharmacies, or even clinic waiting rooms. Make sure the information is readable and interesting, and that your point is made utilizing enticing images and simple words.

5. Hosting Plant Swaps and Herbal Study Groups

Set up plant exchanges or study groups focused on herbs so that locals may share information, plants, and seeds. These events provide fantastic chances to learn and form bonds with others. Encourage others to provide their own insights and advice to create a cooperative atmosphere.

Workshops are a great, practical method to inform and involve your community. They offer a controlled setting where individuals may pick up useful skills and develop self-assurance when utilizing herbal medicine.

1. Planning Your Workshop

Decide the important subjects to discuss in your session. This might be anything from simple herbal gardening to the creation of particular herbal treatments. Create a thorough schedule that allots time for Q&A sessions, presentations, and hands-on activities. Make sure you have prepared the required supplies and tools in advance.

2. Finding a Venue

Select a location that will be both convenient and welcoming to your attendees. Local gardens, community centers, or even your own backyard might serve as appropriate sites. Make sure the area has the amenities you want for your activities and is big enough to hold the amount of guests you anticipate.

3. Promoting Your Workshop

Use a variety of methods to promote your workshop, including social media, neighborhood bulletin boards, neighborhood newsletters, and word-of-mouth. Give precise details on the workshop's date, time, place, and agenda. More people may join up if early bird discounts or group prices are offered.

4. Conducting the Workshop

Give a quick introduction of yourself and the workshop's goals at the beginning of the session. To improve your presentation, use visual aids like slides, charts, and demonstration materials. Provide participatory exercises to participants, such as plant identification, making remedies, and tastings. Promote dialogue and inquiries to establish a lively learning atmosphere.

5. Providing Take-Home Materials

Provide your attendees with pamphlets or handouts that list the main topics discussed throughout the event. Recipes, plant care manuals, and extra resources for education may all be found in these items. Giving out a starting plant or a tiny sample of a herbal medicine can also make an impression on the recipient.

6. Gathering Feedback

Collect feedback from the attendees after the workshop. A straightforward questionnaire or a conversation in groups might be used for this. By giving you feedback, you may better understand what went well and what needs to be improved for future seminars.

Chapter 12: Advanced Herbal Practices

Combining Herbs for Synergistic Effects

It's not uncommon for the whole to be more than the sum of its parts in the field of herbal therapy. A key concept in sophisticated herbal medicines is synergy. Combining several herbs can increase their therapeutic effects, lessen any potential drawbacks, and provide a more comprehensive approach to health and wellbeing.

Understanding Synergy in Herbal Medicine

The combined effects of two or more herbs may be stronger than the individual ones. We call this synergy. This concept has been a component of traditional medicine for many years, appearing in everything from modern phytotherapy to ancient Chinese and Ayurvedic treatments. Comprehending the interrelationships between different plants can enable you to create effective herbal remedies that target an array of medical conditions.

Principles of Combining Herbs

1. **Complementary Actions**: Select botanicals with complementing medicinal properties. For instance, during the cold and flu season, combining an anti-inflammatory herb with an immune-boosting herb can help and relieve symptoms.

2. **Balance and Moderation**: Make sure the mixture stays in check and doesn't overburden the body's systems. The correct combination of herbs may create harmony; some can be relaxing, while others might be energizing.

3. **Potentiation**: Make sure the mixture stays in check and doesn't overburden the body's systems. The correct combination of herbs may create harmony; some can be relaxing, while others might be energizing.

4. **Safety First**: Every time you combine herbs, especially ones with different safety profiles, keep that in mind. Recognize possible interactions and

contraindications, especially for those who are taking medication or have pre-existing medical issues.

Popular Synergistic Herbal Combinations

- **Immune Support Blend**: Echinacea, Elderberry, and Astragalus

    - **Echinacea** boosts immune function and reduces inflammation.

    - **Elderberry** provides antiviral properties.

    - **Astragalus** strengthens overall vitality and immune resilience.

- **Digestive Harmony Blend**: Peppermint, Ginger, and Fennel

    - **Peppermint** soothes the digestive tract and reduces spasms.

    - **Ginger** aids in digestion and alleviates nausea.

o **Fennel** eases bloating and gas.

- **Relaxation and Sleep Blend**: Valerian, Chamomile, and Lemon Balm

  o **Valerian** helps people unwind and get better sleep..

  o **Chamomile** calms the nervous system.

  o **Lemon Balm** reduces anxiety and stress.

Exploring Lesser-Known Medicinal Plants

While many are familiar with popular medicinal herbs like lavender, chamomile, and peppermint, there is a vast world of lesser-known plants with potent therapeutic properties. Delving into these hidden gems can expand your herbal repertoire and provide unique solutions for various health concerns.

Uncommon Medicinal Herbs

1. **Skullcap (Scutellaria lateriflora)**

- o **Uses**: This North American herb is known for its calming effects on the nervous system. It can help with anxiety, insomnia, and stress-related headaches.

- o **Preparation**: Typically used as a tincture or tea.

2. **Holy Basil (Ocimum sanctum)**

- o **Uses**: Also known as Tulsi, Holy Basil is revered in Ayurvedic medicine for its adaptogenic properties, helping the body cope with stress and support overall well-being.

- o **Preparation**: Commonly used in teas, tinctures, and as a culinary herb.

3. **Wood Betony (Stachys officinalis)**

- o **Uses**: Traditionally used in European herbalism, Wood Betony supports nervous system health, digestive issues, and headaches.

- o **Preparation**: Best used as a tea or tincture.

4. **Elecampane (Inula helenium)**

- o **Uses**: Known for its respiratory benefits, Elecampane can help with bronchitis, coughs, and other lung conditions.

- o **Preparation**: Often used in syrups, teas, and tinctures.

5. **Gotu Kola (Centella asiatica)**

- o **Uses**: An important herb in both Ayurvedic and Traditional Chinese Medicine, Gotu Kola supports cognitive function, skin health, and circulatory health.

- o **Preparation**: Can be used in teas, tinctures, and topical preparations.

Integrating Lesser-Known Herbs into Your Practice

Exploring and integrating lesser-known medicinal plants into your practice can be rewarding and beneficial. To get started, follow these steps:

1. **Research**: Learn about the herb's traditional uses, active constituents, and potential health benefits. Reliable sources include herbal medicine books, scientific studies, and reputable herbalists.

2. **Start Small**: Begin with small doses to gauge how the herb affects you or those you are treating. Keep an eye out for any negative drug interactions or reactions.

3. **Grow Your Own**: Many lesser-known medicinal plants can be grown in your garden. This strengthens your bond with the plants and guarantees a continuous supply.

4. **Consult Experts**: Engage with experienced herbalists or join herbalist communities to exchange knowledge and experiences.

5. **Document Your Experience**: Record your observations, plans, and results in a diary. This can help you fine-tune your strategy and be a useful tool for later use.

CHAPTER 13: SUSTAINABLE AND ETHICAL HERBAL GARDENING

Practicing Sustainability in Your Herbal Garden

Sustainable gardening isn't just about growing plants; it's about creating a harmonious environment where both the gardener and the garden thrive. By implementing sustainable practices, you can ensure that your herbal garden remains productive and healthy for years to come while minimizing your environmental footprint.

1. Choosing Native Plants: One of the cornerstones of sustainable gardening is the selection of native plants. These plants are adapted to your local climate and soil conditions, which means they require less water, fertilizer, and pest control. Native plants also support local wildlife, including pollinators like bees and butterflies, which are essential for a healthy ecosystem.

2. Composting: Composting is an excellent way to recycle organic waste and enrich your soil. By composting kitchen scraps, garden clippings, and leaves, you can create nutrient-rich humus that improves soil structure, retains moisture, and provides essential nutrients to your plants. Moreover, composting lessens the need for synthetic fertilizers, which may be bad for the environment.

3. Water Conservation: Water is a precious resource, and conserving it is crucial for sustainable gardening. Implementing drip irrigation systems, using rain barrels, and mulching can significantly reduce water usage. By delivering water straight to the roots of the plants, drip irrigation lowers runoff and evaporation. Rain barrels collect and store rainwater for later use, while mulching helps retain soil moisture and suppress weeds.

4. Organic Pest Control: Avoid chemical pesticides and opt for organic methods to control pests. Encourage beneficial insects, such as ladybugs and predatory wasps, which feed on harmful pests. Planting companion plants can also deter pests; for example, marigolds repel aphids and nematodes. Additionally, using natural remedies like neem oil or insecticidal soap can effectively manage pest problems without harming the environment.

5. Soil Health: A sustainable garden starts with healthy soil. Test your soil frequently to determine its pH and nutrient levels. Add organic materials, such old manure or compost, to your soil to enhance its fertility and structure. To stop soil erosion and lessen the accumulation of pests and diseases, rotate your crops and steer clear of monocultures.

Ethical Wildcrafting: Harvesting Wild Herbs Responsibly

Wildcrafting, the practice of harvesting wild plants for medicinal use, can be a rewarding and sustainable way to source herbs. However, it's essential to approach wildcrafting with respect and responsibility to ensure the long-term health of wild plant populations and their ecosystems.

1. Know Your Plants: Before you begin wildcrafting, make sure you can accurately identify the plants you intend to harvest. Misidentification can lead to the collection of the wrong species, some of which may be endangered or toxic. Invest in a good field guide or take a course on plant identification to enhance your knowledge.

2. Harvesting Ethically: Always follow ethical guidelines when harvesting wild herbs. Never take more than you need, and leave enough plants behind to ensure the population can regenerate. A general rule of thumb is to harvest no more than 10% of a plant population in any given area. Avoid harvesting entire plants; instead, take only the parts you need, such as leaves, flowers, or seeds.

3. Protecting Habitats: Respect the habitats where wild plants grow. Avoid trampling delicate ecosystems and be mindful of your impact on the environment. Follow designated routes to prevent upsetting wildlife. If a plant is growing in a fragile or threatened habitat, consider finding an alternative source or growing it in your garden instead.

4. Legal Considerations: Be aware of the legal regulations regarding wildcrafting in your area. Some plants may be protected by law, and harvesting them without permission can lead to legal consequences. Respect private property borders and always get the required licenses.

5. Sustainable Harvesting Techniques: Use sustainable harvesting techniques to minimize harm to the plants and their surroundings. For example, when harvesting bark, take small sections from different trees rather than stripping bark from one tree. When collecting roots, replant a portion of the root to allow the plant to regenerate. These practices help maintain healthy plant populations and ensure their availability for future generations.

6. Wildcrafting Ethics: Wildcrafting is as much about ethics as it is about technique. Approach the practice with gratitude and respect for the plants and the land. Recognize the customs and wisdom of the native peoples who have been caring for these plants for ages. Consider giving back to the environment by participating in conservation efforts or supporting organizations that protect wild habitats.

CHAPTER 14: HERBAL MEDICINE FOR FAMILIES

Safe Herbs for Children and the Elderly

Herbal medicine offers a natural, gentle approach to health and wellness that can benefit individuals of all ages. When it comes to children and the elderly, special considerations are necessary to ensure safety and efficacy. These populations often require milder, more carefully dosed treatments due to their sensitive systems. The following are some secure herbs that work well for both young people and the elderly:

1. **Chamomile (Matricaria chamomilla)**

   o **Benefits:** Famous for its ability to calm and soothe, chamomile. It is excellent for alleviating anxiety, promoting sleep, and soothing digestive issues.

   o **Usage:** Chamomile tea is a gentle and effective way to introduce this herb to children and the elderly. It's important to ensure that the tea is not too strong and is sweetened if necessary to make it more palatable.

2. **Elderberry (Sambucus nigra)**

   o **Benefits:** Known for its capacity to prevent colds and the flu, elderberries are a potent immune system enhancer. It is rich in vitamins A, B, and C and has strong antiviral properties.

   o **Usage:** Elderberry syrup is a popular preparation that can be given to children and the elderly to strengthen their immune systems, especially during the cold and flu season.

3. **Ginger (Zingiber officinale)**

   o **Benefits:** Ginger is excellent for easing nausea, improving digestion, and relieving joint pain. It has anti-inflammatory and antioxidant properties.

- o **Usage:** Ginger tea, made by steeping fresh ginger slices in hot water, is a gentle remedy that can be used for digestive issues and joint pain relief. For children, ensure the tea is mild and sweetened with honey or sugar.

4. Lavender (Lavandula angustifolia)

- o **Benefits:** Lavender is known for its relaxing and calming effects. It can help with sleep problems, anxiety, and stress.

- o **Usage:** Lavender essential oil can be used in a diffuser to promote relaxation and improve sleep. Lavender sachets can also be placed under pillows to help children and the elderly sleep better.

5. Peppermint (Mentha piperita)

- o **Benefits:** Peppermint is effective for soothing digestive issues, reducing headaches, and alleviating congestion.

- o **Usage:** Peppermint tea is a safe and gentle option for children and the elderly to ease digestive discomfort. A few drops of peppermint oil in a steam inhalation can help with congestion.

Integrating Herbal Medicine into Family Health

Integrating herbal medicine into your family's health regimen involves more than just choosing the right herbs. It requires an understanding of how to incorporate these remedies into daily routines, ensuring that they are used safely and effectively. Here are some strategies to seamlessly integrate herbal medicine into family health:

1. **Start with Familiar Herbs**

   - o Begin by introducing herbs that are well-known and commonly used, such as chamomile, peppermint, and ginger. These herbs are generally well-tolerated and can be easily incorporated into everyday meals and beverages.

2. **Create a Family Herbal Medicine Cabinet**

   o Designate a space in your home for storing herbal medicines, such as dried herbs, tinctures, salves, and essential oils. Ensure that all family members know where to find these remedies and how to use them.

3. **Educate Your Family**

   o Take the time to educate your family about the benefits and uses of different herbs. Understanding how and why herbal remedies work can encourage more consistent and confident use.

4. **Incorporate Herbs into Daily Routines**

o Make herbal teas a regular part of your family's daily routine. For example, a cup of chamomile tea before bed can become a comforting nightly ritual. Adding ginger to meals or using peppermint oil in a diffuser can be simple ways to integrate herbs into everyday life.

5. Use Herbal Remedies for Common Ailments

o For minor health issues such as colds, digestive problems, or stress, reach for herbal remedies first. Having a go-to herbal solution for common ailments can reduce the need for over-the-counter medications and foster a more holistic approach to health.

6. Consult with a Professional

o If you are new to herbal medicine or are dealing with specific health concerns, consider consulting with a qualified herbalist or naturopath. They can provide personalized advice and help you create a tailored herbal regimen for your family.

7. Practice Safe Dosing

- Pay careful attention to dosing, especially for children and the elderly. Start with little doses and keep an eye out for any negative effects. Adjust dosages as needed based on the individual's response to the herb.

8. Grow Your Own Herbs

- You could think about planting a small herb garden to produce your own healing plants. This can be a rewarding family project and ensures a fresh, organic supply of herbs. Teach children about gardening and the medicinal properties of plants to foster a lifelong appreciation for natural remedies.

CHAPTER 15: MODERN APPLICATIONS OF HERBAL MEDICINE

Using Herbs in the Digital Age

Our lives have been completely transformed by the internet era, and this includes how we get and apply herbal medicine. Technology today offers previously unheard-of possibilities for studying, discussing, and using herbal medicine. For novices and seasoned herbalists alike, the digital world provides a multitude of tools, including virtual groups and online courses.

1. Online Learning and Resources

It's never been simpler to learn about herbal medicine thanks to the internet's emergence. There are a plethora of online resources that include workshops, webinars, and courses for varying skill levels. Online learning platforms such as Coursera, Udemy, and other specialist herbal medicine sites provide extensive courses ranging from fundamental plant identification to sophisticated herbal synthesis.

2. Mobile Apps

For herbal fans, mobile applications have also developed into useful resources. While some apps, like "HerbList" and "iPlant," provide comprehensive information on the uses, advantages, and possible drawbacks of different herbs, others, like "PlantSnap" and "iHerbarium," assist users in identifying plants using their cellphones. It's simple to have a plethora of herbal information in your pocket with these applications.

3. Social Media and Online Communities

Herbal medicine lovers are active participants in thriving groups on social media sites like Facebook, Instagram, and Reddit. These communities offer a forum for inquiries, advice, and experience sharing. Being a part of these groups may provide inspiration, motivation, and support from like-minded people.

4. E-Books and Digital Libraries

Digital libraries and e-books are great tools for getting access to material on herbal medicine. There is a huge selection of books available on sites like Kindle, Google Books, and different online libraries for herbal medicine. This facilitates keeping up with the most recent findings and industry trends.

Research and Innovations in Herbal Medicine

Herbal medicine is a discipline that is always changing due to new methods and continuous study. Many of the traditional uses of herbs have been validated by modern research, and new uses are being found on a regular basis.

1. Scientific Validation

Many investigations have been carried out recently to formally confirm the effectiveness of certain plants. For instance, several studies have confirmed the anti-inflammatory qualities of turmeric (Curcuma longa), supporting its historic usage in the treatment of inflammation. Analogously, studies have confirmed the adaptogenic qualities of ashwagandha (Withania somnifera), hence endorsing its application in the treatment of stress.

2. Integrative Medicine

Integrative medicine is becoming more and more well-liked. It blends traditional Western medicine with supplementary therapies like herbal medicine. This method acknowledges the importance of both contemporary and traditional methods for advancing health and wellbeing. Practitioners of integrative medicine frequently combine herbs with prescription drugs to improve therapeutic results and lessen negative effects.

3. Personalized Herbal Medicine

The development of customized herbal medicine has been made possible by developments in genetics and biotechnology. Healthcare professionals can customise herbal therapies for each patient by knowing their genetic composition. Herbal therapies become safer and more successful with this tailored approach.

4. New Extraction and Formulation Techniques

The potency and usefulness of herbal medications have increased due to advancements in extraction and formulation processes. Supercritical fluid extraction and nano-formulation are two contemporary techniques that improve the bioavailability and efficacy of herbal components. These developments guarantee that patients get the most out of their herbal remedies.

5. Sustainable and Ethical Sourcing

The need for ethical and ecological herb procurement is growing along with the demand for herbal treatment. Novel approaches to cultivation, such organic farming and wildcrafting, contribute to the assurance that herbs are cultivated and collected in a way that respects the environment and human rights. This helps local populations maintain their standard of living while also protecting the biodiversity of therapeutic plants.

6. Herbal Medicine and Mental Health

One important contemporary use of herbal medicine is the realization of the potential benefits of using herbs in the treatment of mental illness. More and more people are turning to herbs like valerian (Valeriana officinalis) and St. John's Wort (Hypericum perforatum) to treat ailments like anxiety and depression. The potential of herbs to help mental health is still being investigated.

7. Global Collaboration and Knowledge Sharing

The recognition of the possible advantages of employing herbs to treat mental disease is a significant modern use of herbal therapy. Herbs like St. John's Wort (Hypericum perforatum) and valerian (Valeriana officinalis) are being used by an increasing number of individuals to treat conditions including depression and anxiety. Research is currently ongoing to determine whether herbs might improve mental health.

CONCLUSION

The Future of Herbal Medicine

Since plants were the main source of healing in prehistoric societies, herbal medicine has played a significant role in human history. Herbal medicine is positioned to have a big impact on healthcare in the future given the current interest in natural and holistic approaches to health. Herbal therapy is becoming more widely accepted and incorporated into conventional healthcare as research from contemporary science supports the effectiveness of many traditional treatments.

The possibility of individualized herbal therapies is one of the most promising developments in herbal therapy. Advances in genetics and biotechnology are opening the door to more precise and customized approaches to health and well-being. Imagine a day when the particular herbs chosen for your individual needs may be determined by your genetic profile. This degree of customization may lower the possibility of negative responses and increase the efficacy of herbal treatments.

The preservation and production of therapeutic plants is another exciting field. There's a focused effort to conserve natural areas and endangered plant species as people become more conscious of the value of biodiversity and sustainable practices. Modern agricultural methods, such hydroponics and vertical gardening, are being used to cultivate medicinal herbs in urban settings so that city dwellers can have easier access to them.

Moreover, the combination of digital health technology and herbal medicine is poised to completely transform our understanding of wellbeing. Online resources and mobile apps may track health outcomes, provide individualized suggestions, and offer real-time help on the usage of herbal treatments. People may take charge of their health and make educated decisions about their herbal medication regimens with the help of this digital support.

Continuing Your Journey in Herbal Healing

You are just getting started on your adventure into the field of herbal medicine. Always keep in mind that the world of medicinal herbs is dynamic and ever-changing as you research and cultivate your own. Finding a new herb, perfecting a new preparation method, or learning a new facet of plant biology—there's always something new to learn.

To assist you in advancing on your herbal healing path, consider the following steps:

1. **Stay Informed**: Keep up with the latest research and developments in herbal medicine. Subscribe to journals, join online forums, and attend workshops and conferences. The more you know, the more effective and safe your practice will be.

2. **Experiment and Document**: Don't be afraid to experiment with different herbs and preparation methods. Keep a detailed journal of your experiences, noting the effects of different

remedies and any adjustments you make. This will help you refine your practice over time.

3. **Connect with Others**: Build a community of like-minded individuals who share your interest in herbal medicine. Exchange knowledge, exchange stories and offer mutual encouragement. This sense of community can be incredibly enriching and motivating.

4. **Educate Yourself**: Consider taking formal courses in herbal medicine. Many institutions offer programs ranging from short courses to full certifications. This structured learning can deepen your understanding and open up new opportunities.

5. **Practice Mindfulness**: Herbal medicine is as much about the journey as it is about the destination. Take time to connect with the plants you grow, understand their life cycles, and appreciate the role they play in the ecosystem. This

mindful approach can enhance your overall experience and deepen your connection to nature.

6. **Advocate for Herbal Medicine**: Share your knowledge and experiences with others. Write blogs, give talks, or volunteer to teach classes. Advocacy can help spread the benefits of herbal medicine and contribute to its acceptance and integration into mainstream healthcare.

9 7 9 8 3 3 4 1 8 8 9 3 8